STRONG BONES, HEALTHY MEALS

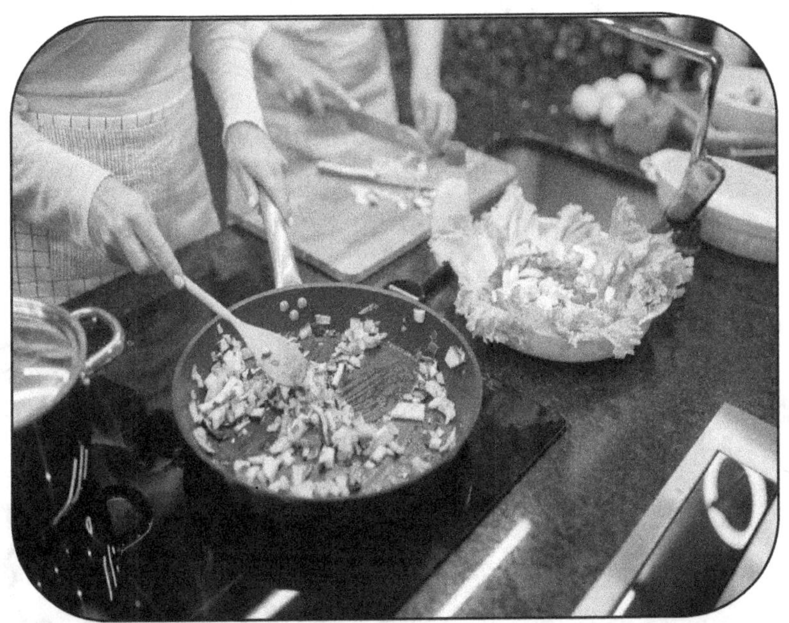

A Comprehensive Osteoporosis Diet Cookbook for Seniors with Delicious Recipes to Nourish and Reduce Fraction

MELISSA D. JOHNSON

1 Melissa D. Johnson

COPYRIGHTS

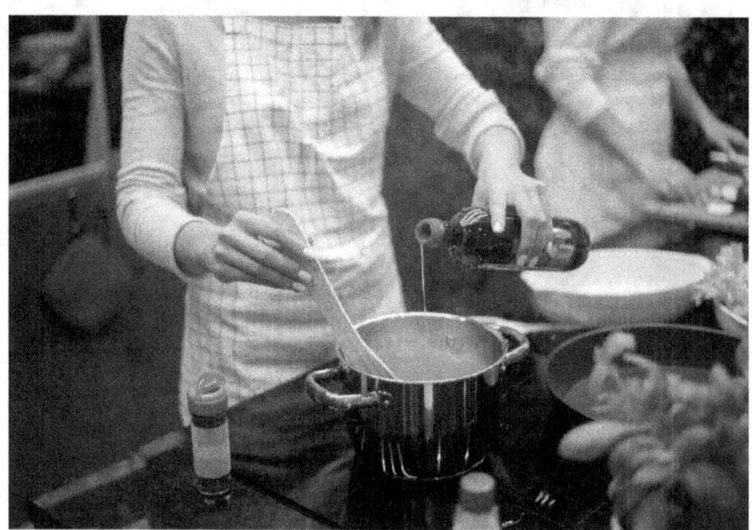

CONTENTS

Introduction 5

Understanding Osteoporosis and the Power of Diet 7

Benefits of a Bone-Healthy Eating Plan 9

Chapter 1 11

30-Recipes 11

Chapter 2: 29

15-Vitamin D Duos: Pairing Foods Rich in Vitamin D & Calcium 29

Chapter 3 49

Protein Power: Essential for Bone Health and Muscle Maintenance 49

Chapter 4 62

Chapter 6 70

30-Breakfast Recipes To support a healthy bone for your family or yourself 70

Chapter 7 85

20-Lunchtime: Easy and Nutritious Options for Seniors 85

some convenient lunch options for people at work who may not have time to cook, along with stores where they can purchase them immediately 88

Chapter 8 96

Dinnertime Delectables: Satisfying and Bone-Building Main Courses 96

Chapter 9 108

Sweet Endings: Healthy and Delicious Desserts for Seniors 108

Conclusion 115

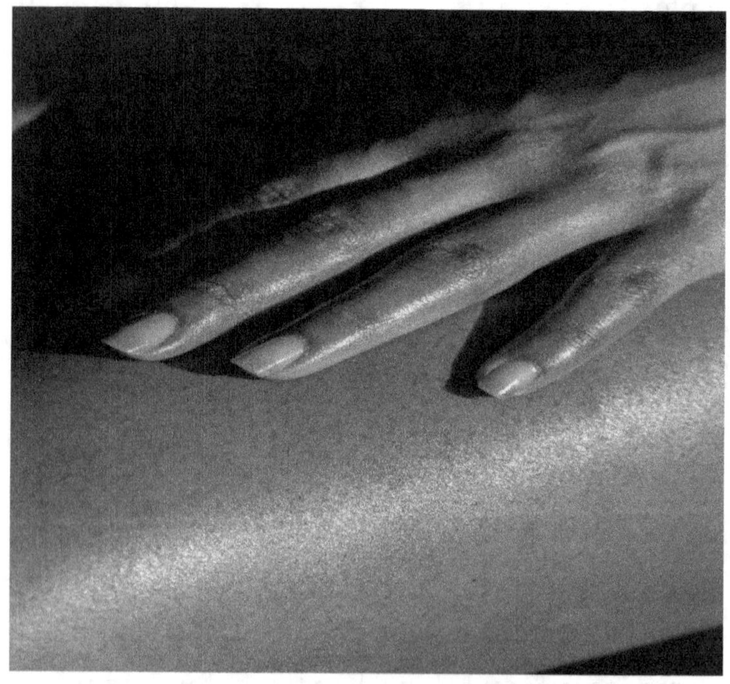

INTRODUCTION

Osteoporosis. The word itself sounds heavy, doesn't it? That weight hit me hard when my dear aunt, all the way from Germany, landed unexpectedly in the hospital where I work - me, Dr. Melissa D. Johnson. There was no warning, just a frantic call followed by a worried entourage wheeling her in.

Tests revealed the culprit: weak bones. The doctors prescribed a regimen of medication, but seeing my aunt, barely 50, facing a future reliant on drugs just didn't sit right with me. There had to be another way.

That's when I remembered my passion for food and its incredible power to heal. Meals weren't just sustenance; they were building blocks, bricks and mortar for our bodies. So, I rolled up my sleeves and got to work in my kitchen.

The result? A symphony of flavors, a colorful kaleidoscope of fruits, vegetables, and proteins, all designed to nourish and strengthen bones. It was more than just food; it was a plan, a delicious rebellion against the limitations osteoporosis tried to impose.

And then, the magic happened. Within just six days of following this new way of eating, the change in my aunt was undeniable. Her energy levels soared, her steps became lighter, and her smile brighter. It was a testament to the power of food as medicine.

News of her transformation traveled fast. Back in Germany, my aunt became her own advocate, referring friends facing similar challenges to my hospital. Now, I want to share that same power with you.

No matter your age or diagnosis, these meals can be your allies in living a healthy, active life. So, grab your apron, turn the page, and let's go.

Understanding Osteoporosis and the Power of Diet

Our bones, the silent supporters beneath our skin, are a marvel of living tissue. Constantly remodeling and rebuilding themselves, they grant us structure, support our movement, and protect our vital organs. But sometimes, this intricate process goes awry, leading to a condition called osteoporosis.

Osteoporosis, literally meaning "porous bone," weakens bone density, making them more susceptible to fractures. Often dubbed the "silent thief" because it often progresses without symptoms until a fracture occurs, osteoporosis can be a significant concern, especially for seniors.

But here's the good news: While osteoporosis can't be reversed, it can be managed. And a powerful tool in this fight? Your diet!

Food is more than just fuel; it's a treasure trove of essential nutrients that our bodies crave to function optimally. For bone health, certain nutrients are absolute champions:

Calcium: The building block of bones, calcium provides the foundation for strong, dense bone tissue.

Vitamin D: Often called the "sunshine vitamin," Vitamin D helps your body absorb calcium effectively. Think of it as the key that unlocks the calcium treasure chest!

Protein: A crucial building block for bones and muscles, protein helps maintain bone strength and supports mobility.

Vitamin K: Often overlooked, Vitamin K plays a vital role in bone metabolism, ensuring proper calcium utilization.

Fruits & Vegetables: Packed with antioxidants and essential vitamins, fruits and vegetables contribute to overall bone health and well-being.

This cookbook is your guide to harnessing the power of these bone-building nutrients. We'll explore delicious recipes rich in calcium, Vitamin D, protein, and other essential elements. We'll delve into the importance of a balanced diet and guide you in making informed choices that support strong, healthy bones.

Benefits of a Bone-Healthy Eating Plan

Building strong bones is undoubtedly the primary focus of this cookbook, but the benefits of a bone-healthy eating plan extend far beyond your skeletal system. Here's how this delicious approach to food can nourish your entire well-being:

Overall Health Boost: A diet rich in calcium, Vitamin D, protein, and essential vitamins translates to a stronger, healthier you. You may experience improved energy levels, a stronger immune system, and better resistance to chronic illnesses.

Muscle Maintenance: Protein, a key component of a bone-healthy diet, also plays a vital role in muscle health. By incorporating protein-rich foods, you can support muscle strength and function, promoting better balance and reducing the risk of falls.

Improved Heart Health: Many bone-healthy foods, like fruits, vegetables, and fish, are also heart-healthy superstars. This dietary approach can help lower blood pressure, regulate cholesterol levels, and reduce your risk of heart disease.

Weight Management: By focusing on whole, unprocessed foods with a balanced mix of nutrients, you'll feel fuller for longer, promoting healthy weight management. This can have a ripple effect on your overall health, including reducing stress on your joints and bones.

Enhanced Mood: Eating a well-balanced diet rich in essential vitamins and minerals can positively impact your mood and cognitive function. You may experience increased energy levels, improved focus, and a brighter outlook.

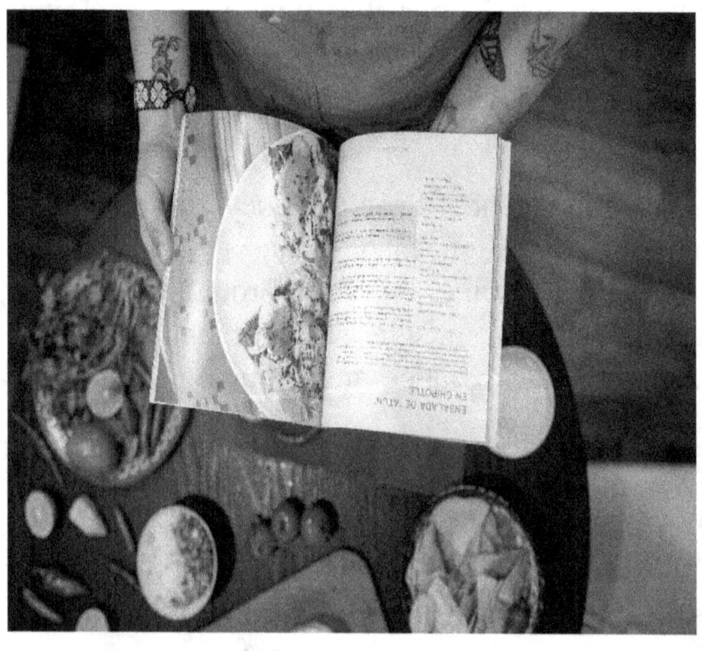

CHAPTER 1

30-Recipes

1. **Calcium-Rich Breakfast Smoothie**
   - **Ingredients**: 1 cup kale, 1/2 cup plain yogurt, 1 banana, 1/2 cup orange juice, 1/4 cup almonds.
   - **Preparation:** Blend all ingredients until smooth. Serve chilled.
   - **Where to get it:** Local grocery store or farmers' market.
   - **Nutritional Value:** High in calcium, vitamin C, and protein.
2. **Spinach and Mushroom Omelette**
   - **Ingredients:** 2 eggs, 1 cup spinach, 1/2 cup sliced mushrooms, 1/4 cup shredded cheese.
   - **Preparation:** Whisk eggs, then pour into a pan over medium heat. Add spinach and mushrooms, cook until eggs are set. Sprinkle cheese and fold over.

- **Where to get it:** Local grocery store.
- **Nutritional Value:** Rich in calcium, vitamin D, and protein.

3. **Salmon Salad**
    - Ingredients: 4 oz grilled salmon, mixed greens, cherry tomatoes, cucumber slices, 1 tbsp olive oil, lemon juice.
    - **Preparation:** Arrange greens, tomatoes, and cucumbers on a plate. Top with grilled salmon. Drizzle olive oil and lemon juice.
    - **Where to get it:** Local fish market and grocery store.
    - **Nutritional Value:** High in omega-3 fatty acids, calcium, and vitamin K.

4. **Quinoa and Vegetable Stir-Fry**
   - **Ingredients:** 1 cup cooked quinoa, mixed vegetables (bell peppers, broccoli, carrots), 2 tbsp soy sauce, 1 tbsp sesame oil.
   - **Preparation:** Sauté vegetables in sesame oil until tender. Add cooked quinoa and soy sauce, and stir until heated through.
   - **Where to get it:** Local grocery store.
   - Nutritional Value: High in calcium, protein, and fiber.

5. **Greek Yogurt Parfait**
   - Ingredients: Greek yogurt, mixed berries, granola.
   - Preparation: Layer yogurt, berries, and granola in a glass. Repeat layers.
   - **Where to get it:** Local grocery store.
   - **Nutritional Value:** Rich in calcium, vitamin C, and protein.

6. **Tofu and Vegetable Stir-Fry**
   - **Ingredients:** 1 cup tofu, mixed vegetables (broccoli, bell peppers, snap peas), 2 tbsp soy sauce, 1 tbsp sesame oil.
   - **Preparation**: Sauté tofu and vegetables in sesame oil until tender. Add soy sauce and stir until heated through.
   - **Where to get it:** Local grocery store.
   - **Nutritional Value:** High in calcium, protein, and vitamin K.
7. **Berry Spinach Salad**
   - **Ingredients:** Spinach, mixed berries, feta cheese, walnuts, balsamic vinaigrette.
   - **Preparation:** Toss spinach, berries, cheese, and walnuts in a bowl. Drizzle with balsamic vinaigrette.
   - **Where to get it:** Local grocery store or farmers' market.
   - **Nutritional Value:** Rich in calcium, vitamin C, and antioxidants.

8. **Sweet Potato and Black Bean Burrito**
    - **Ingredients:** Whole wheat tortilla, sweet potato, black beans, avocado, salsa.
    - **Preparation:** Fill the tortilla with mashed sweet potato, black beans, avocado, and salsa. Roll up and serve.
    - **Where to get it:** Local grocery store.
    - **Nutritional Value:** High in calcium, fiber, and vitamin A.

9. **Broccoli and Cheese Soup**
    - **Ingredients:** Broccoli, onion, garlic, vegetable broth, cheddar cheese, milk.
    - **Preparation:** Sauté onion and garlic, add broccoli and broth. Simmer until tender, then blend until smooth. Stir in cheese and milk.
    - **Where to get it:** Local grocery store.

- **Nutritional Value:** Rich in calcium, vitamin C, and protein.

10. **Chia Seed Pudding**
    - **Ingredients:** Chia seeds, almond milk, honey, vanilla extract.
    - **Preparation:** Mix chia seeds, almond milk, honey, and vanilla extract in a jar. Refrigerate overnight.
    - **Where to get it:** Local grocery store.
    - **Nutritional Value:** High in calcium, fiber, and omega-3 fatty acids.

11. **Chicken and Vegetable Skewers**
    - **Ingredients:** Chicken breast, bell peppers, zucchini, cherry tomatoes, olive oil, Italian seasoning.
    - **Preparation:** Thread chicken and vegetables onto skewers. Brush with olive oil and sprinkle with seasoning. Grill until cooked through.
    - **Where to get it:** Local grocery store.

- **Nutritional Value:** High in protein, vitamin C, and calcium.

12. **Mango Avocado Smoothie**
    - **Ingredients**: Mango, avocado, spinach, almond milk, honey.
    - **Preparation:** Blend all ingredients until smooth. Serve chilled.
    - **Where to get it:** Local grocery store or farmers' market.
    - **Nutritional Value:** Rich in calcium, vitamin C, and healthy fats.

13. **Turkey and Vegetable Stir-Fry**
    - **Ingredients:** Turkey breast, mixed vegetables (snow peas, carrots, bell peppers), soy sauce, garlic, ginger.
    - **Preparation:** Sauté turkey and vegetables in garlic and ginger until cooked. Add soy sauce and stir until heated through.
    - **Where to get it:** Local grocery store.
    - **Nutritional Value:** High in protein, calcium, and vitamin C.

14. **Quinoa Salad with Cranberries and Almonds**
   - **Ingredients:** Cooked quinoa, dried cranberries, sliced almonds, spinach, lemon juice, olive oil.
   - Preparation: Mix quinoa, cranberries, almonds, and spinach in a bowl. Drizzle with lemon juice and olive oil.
   - Where to get it: Local grocery store.
   - Nutritional Value: Rich in calcium, protein, and antioxidants.

15. **Tuna Salad Wrap**
   - **Ingredients:** Canned tuna, whole wheat wrap, mixed greens, cucumber slices, Greek yogurt, Dijon mustard.
   - **Preparation:** Mix tuna, Greek yogurt, and Dijon mustard. Spread onto the wrap, add greens and cucumber. Roll up and serve.
   - **Where to get it:** Local grocery store.

- **Nutritional Value:** High in protein, calcium, and omega-3 fatty acids.

16. **Oatmeal with Almond Butter and Banana**
    - Ingredients: Rolled oats, almond butter, banana, honey.
    - Preparation: Cook oats according to package instructions. Top with almond butter, and sliced banana, and drizzle with honey.
    - Where to get it: Local grocery store.
    - Nutritional Value: Rich in calcium, fiber, and protein.

17. **Eggplant and Tomato Bake**
    - **Ingredients:** Eggplant, tomatoes, garlic, olive oil, basil, mozzarella cheese.
    - **Preparation:** Layer sliced eggplant and tomatoes in a baking dish. Drizzle with olive oil, sprinkle with minced garlic and basil. Top with mozzarella cheese. Bake until tender.

- **Where to get it:** Local grocery store.
- **Nutritional Value:** High in calcium, vitamin C, and antioxidants.

18. **Lentil Soup**
    - Ingredients: Lentils, onion, carrots, celery,

, garlic, vegetable broth, cumin, turmeric.

- **Preparation:** Sauté onion, carrots, celery, and garlic until softened. Add lentils, vegetable broth, cumin, and turmeric. Simmer until lentils are tender.
- **Where to get it:** Local grocery store.
- **Nutritional Value:** High in protein, fiber, and iron.

19. **Mushroom and Spinach Stuffed Chicken Breast**
   - **Ingredients:** Chicken breast, mushrooms, spinach, garlic, Parmesan cheese.
   - **Preparation:** Flatten chicken breast, then top with sautéed mushrooms, spinach, garlic, and Parmesan cheese. Roll up and secure with toothpicks. Bake until cooked through.
   - **Where to get it:** Local grocery store.
   - **Nutritional Value:** Rich in protein, calcium, and vitamin D.

20. **Greek Salad with Grilled Chicken**
   - **Ingredients:** Grilled chicken breast, mixed greens, cucumber, cherry tomatoes, red onion, Kalamata olives, feta cheese, olive oil, lemon juice.

   Preparation: Toss greens, cucumber, tomatoes, onion, olives, and feta cheese in a bowl.

- Top with grilled chicken. Drizzle with olive oil and lemon juice.
- **Where to get it:** Local grocery store.
- **Nutritional Value:** High in protein, calcium, and antioxidants.

21. **Stuffed Bell Peppers**
- **Ingredients:** Bell peppers, quinoa, black beans, corn, diced tomatoes, chili powder, cumin, shredded cheese.
- **Preparation:** Cut tops off bell peppers and remove seeds.
- Mix cooked quinoa, black beans, corn, diced tomatoes, chili powder, and cumin.
- Stuff peppers with mixture, top with shredded cheese. Bake until peppers are done.
- **Where to get it:** Local grocery store.
- **Nutritional Value:** Rich in calcium, fiber, and vitamin C.

22. **Cauliflower Rice Stir-Fry**
   - **Ingredients:** Cauliflower, mixed vegetables (peas, carrots, bell peppers), eggs, soy sauce.
   - **Preparation:** Pulse cauliflower in a food processor to resemble rice. Sauté mixed vegetables in a pan, then add cauliflower rice.
   - Put vegetables to one side, scramble eggs on the other side. Mix together and add soy sauce.
   - **Where to get it:** Local grocery store.
   - **Nutritional Value:** High in calcium, fiber, and vitamin C.
23. **Almond-Crusted Baked Cod**
   - **Ingredients:** Cod fillets, almond meal, lemon zest, garlic powder, paprika, olive oil.
   - **Preparation:** Mix almond meal, lemon zest, garlic powder, and paprika. Coat cod fillets with mixture and drizzle with olive oil. Bake until fish is cooked through.

- **Where to get it:** Local fish market or grocery store.
- Nutritional Value: Rich in omega-3 fatty acids, calcium, and protein.

24. **Mango Spinach Salad with Grilled Shrimp**

- **Ingredients:** Mango, spinach, red onion, grilled shrimp, avocado, lime juice, olive oil.
- **Preparation:** Toss spinach, mango, onion, and avocado in a bowl.
- Top with grilled shrimp. Drizzle with lime juice and olive oil.
- **Where to get it:** Local grocery store.
- **Nutritional Value:** High in protein, calcium, and vitamin C.

25. **Vegetable and Bean Soup**
   - **Ingredients:** Mixed vegetables (carrots, celery, onion, potatoes), vegetable broth, kidney beans, green beans, diced tomatoes, Italian seasoning.
   - **Preparation:** Sauté vegetables until softened.
   - Add vegetable broth, beans, tomatoes, and seasoning.
   - Simmer until vegetables are d
   - **Where to get it:** Local grocery store.
   - **Nutritional Value:** Rich in calcium, fiber, and vitamin C.
26. **Pumpkin and Lentil Curry**
   - Ingredients: Pumpkin, lentils, onion, garlic, ginger, curry powder, coconut milk.
   - Preparation: Sauté onion, garlic, and ginger until fragrant. Add pumpkin, lentils, curry powder, and coconut milk. Simmer until pumpkin and lentils are tender.

- Where to get it: Local grocery store.
- Nutritional Value: High in protein, fiber, and vitamin A.

27. **Turkey and Sweet Potato Chili**
    - **Ingredients:** Ground turkey, sweet potatoes, onion, bell peppers, diced tomatoes, kidney beans, chili powder, cumin.
    - **Preparation:** Brown turkey with onion and bell peppers.
    - Add sweet potatoes, tomatoes, beans, and spices.
    - Simmer the sweet potatoes until its done.
    - **Where to get it:** Local grocery store.
    - **Nutritional Value:** Rich in protein, fiber, and vitamin C.

28. **Broccoli and Cheddar Stuffed Baked Potato**

- Ingredients: Baked potato, steamed broccoli, cheddar cheese, Greek yogurt, chives.
- **Preparation:** Slice open baked potato and fluff insides. Top with steamed broccoli, cheddar cheese, and Greek yogurt. Garnish with chives.
- **Where to get it:** Local grocery store. Check the label
- **Nutritional Value:** High in calcium, vitamin C, and protein.

29. **Chicken and White Bean Soup**

- Ingredients: Chicken breast, white beans, carrots, celery, onion, garlic, chicken broth, thyme.
- Preparation: Sauté onion, carrots, celery, and garlic until softened. Add chicken, beans, broth, and thyme. Simmer until chicken is cooked through.

- Where to get it: Local grocery store.
- Nutritional Value: Rich in protein, fiber, and vitamin C.

30. **Avocado and Tomato Toast**
    - **Ingredients:** Whole grain bread, avocado, tomatoes, feta cheese, basil.
    - **Preparation:** Toast bread, then spread mashed avocado on top. Add sliced tomatoes, crumbled feta cheese, and basil leaves.
    - **Where to get it:** Local grocery store.
    - **Nutritional Value:** High in calcium, vitamin C, and healthy fats.

CHAPTER 2

Vitamin D Duos: Pairing Foods Rich in Vitamin D & Calcium

1. **Grilled Salmon with Steamed Broccoli**
   - Ingredients:
     - 4 oz salmon fillet
     - 1 cup broccoli florets
     - Olive oil
     - Lemon juice
     - Salt and pepper
   - **Preparation:**
     1. Preheat grill to medium-high heat.
     2. Combine salmon with olive oil and season with salt and pepper. Grill for 2-5 minutes on each side, or until cooked through.
     3. Steam broccoli until tender-crisp.
     4. Drizzle salmon with lemon juice before serving.

- **Where to get it:** Local fish market and grocery store.
- **Nutritional Value:** Salmon provides Vitamin D and calcium, while broccoli offers additional calcium and Vitamin C.

2. **Spinach and Mushroom Stuffed Chicken Breast with Quinoa**
   - **Ingredients:**
     - 2 chicken breasts
     - 1 cup cooked quinoa
     - 1 cup spinach, chopped
     - 1/2 cup mushrooms, sliced
     - Garlic powder
     - Olive oil
     - Salt and pepper
   - **Preparation:**
     1. Preheat oven to 375°F (190°C).
     2. In a skillet, sauté spinach and mushrooms with olive oil and garlic powder till. Season it with salt and pepper.

3. Slice a pocket into each chicken breast and stuff with the spinach-mushroom mixture.
4. Place stuffed chicken breasts on a baking dish and bake for 20-30 minutes, or until chicken is done.
5. Serve with already-cooked quinoa.

Where to get it: Local grocery store.

Nutritional Value: Chicken provides protein and Vitamin D, spinach offers calcium, while quinoa adds more calcium and fiber.

3. **Tuna and Avocado Salad with Kale Chips**
   - **Ingredients:**
       - 1 can tuna, drained
       - 1 avocado, diced
       - 2 cups kale leaves
       - Olive oil
       - Lemon juice
       - Salt and pepper

Preparation:

7. In a bowl, mix tuna and diced avocado. Season with salt, pepper, and a splash of lemon juice.
8. Massage kale leaves with olive oil and spread on a baking sheet. Bake at 350°F (175°C) for 10-15 minutes until crispy.
9. Serve tuna and avocado salad with kale chips on the side.

   - **Where to get it:** Local grocery store or fish market.

- **Nutritional Value:** Tuna provides Vitamin D and protein, avocado adds healthy fats and calcium, while kale chips offer calcium and Vitamin K.

4. **Egg and Cheese Breakfast Burrito with Sautéed Spinach**
   - **Ingredients:**
       - 2 large eggs
       - 1/4 cup shredded cheese
       - 1 cup spinach
       - 1 whole wheat tortilla
       - Olive oil
       - Salt and pepper
   - **Preparation:**
       1. Scramble eggs in a pan with olive oil until cooked.
       2. Stir in shredded cheese till melted.
       3. In another pan, sauté spinach with a little olive oil until wilted.

  4. Season it with salt and pepper.
  5. Warm tortilla in the microwave or on a skillet.
  6. Fill tortilla with scrambled eggs and cheese mixture, and top with sautéed spinach.

- **Where to get it:** Local grocery store.
- **Nutritional Value:** Eggs provide Vitamin D and protein, cheese adds calcium, while spinach offers additional calcium and iron.

5. **Mushroom and Swiss Cheese Omelette with Whole Grain Toast**
   - **Ingredients:**
     - 2 eggs
     - 1/4 cup sliced mushrooms
     - 1 slice Swiss cheese
     - 1 slice whole grain bread
     - Olive oil
     - Salt and pepper

- **Preparation:**
    1. In a non-stick skillet, sauté mushrooms with olive oil until golden brown.
    2. Remove from skillet and set aside.
    3. Beat eggs in a bowl and pour into the skillet. Cook until the edges set, then sprinkle sautéed mushrooms on one half of the omelette.
    4. Fold the other half over the mushrooms and cook until the eggs are fully set.
    5. Top omelette with a slice of Swiss cheese and let it melt.
    6. Toast a slice of whole grain bread.
    7. Serve the omelette with whole grain toast on the side.

Where to get it: Local grocery store.
Nutritional Value: Eggs provide Vitamin D and protein, Swiss cheese adds calcium, while whole grain bread offers additional calcium and fiber.

6. **Sardine and Spinach Salad with Orange Vinaigrette**
   - **Ingredients:**
     - 1 can sardines in olive oil
     - 2 cups fresh spinach leaves
     - 1 orange, juiced
     - 1 tablespoon olive oil
     - 1 teaspoon honey
     - Salt and pepper to taste
   - **Preparation:**
     1. Drain sardines and set aside.
     2. In a large bowl, toss spinach leaves with sardines.
     3. In a small bowl, mix together orange juice, olive oil, honey, salt, and pepper to make the vinaigrette.

4. Drizzle the vinaigrette over the salad and toss to coat evenly.

- **Where to get it:** Local grocery store or fish market.
- **Nutritional Value:** Sardines provide Vitamin D and omega-3 fatty acids, spinach adds calcium, while the orange vinaigrette offers additional Vitamin C.

7. **Shrimp and Asparagus Stir-Fry with Brown Rice**

- **Ingredients:**
    - 8 oz shrimp, peeled and deveined
    - 1 bunch asparagus, trimmed and cut into pieces
    - 2 cloves garlic, minced
    - 1 tablespoon soy sauce
    - 1 tablespoon sesame oil
    - Cooked brown rice

Preparation:

- Warm sesame oil in afrying pan on medium heat.
- Put minced garlic and cook until fragrant.
- Add shrimp and cook until pink and cooked through.
- Add asparagus to the skillet and stir-fry until tender-crisp.
- Stir in soy sauce and cook for another minute.
- Serve shrimp and asparagus stir-fry over cooked brown rice.

- **Where to get it:** Local grocery store or fish market.

- **Nutritional Value:** Shrimp provides Vitamin D and protein, asparagus adds calcium, while brown rice offers additional fiber and nutrients.

8. **Cod and Vegetable Packets**
    - **Ingredients:**
        - 2 cod fillets
        - 1 cup cherry tomatoes, halved
        - 1 cup sliced zucchini
        - 1/4 cup sliced red onion
        - 2 tablespoons olive oil
        - 2 tablespoons lemon juice
        - Salt and pepper to taste
    - **Preparation:**
        1. Preheat oven to 375°F (190°C).
        2. Place each cod fillet on a piece of parchment paper. Top with cherry tomatoes, zucchini, and red onion.
        3. Drizzle olive oil and lemon juice over the fish and vegetables. Season with salt and pepper.
        4. Fold parchment paper to create packets and seal tightly.

5. Place packets on a baking sheet and bake for 15-20 minutes, or until fish is cooked through.

- **Where to get it:** Local fish market or grocery store.
- **Nutritional Value:** Cod provides Vitamin D and protein, vegetables add calcium and antioxidants, while the lemon juice adds Vitamin C.

9. **Salmon and Quinoa Salad with Lemon-Herb Dressing**
   - Ingredients:
     - 2 salmon fillets
     - 1 cup cooked quinoa
     - 2 cups mixed greens
       One And four cup chopped fresh herbs (such as parsley, dill, and chives)
     - 2 tablespoons olive oil
     - 1 tablespoon lemon juice
     - Salt and pepper to taste

- **Preparation:**
    1. Season salmon fillets with salt, pepper, and a squeeze of lemon juice. Grill or bake until cooked through.
    2. In a large bowl, combine cooked quinoa, mixed greens, and chopped fresh herbs.
    3. In a small bowl, whisk together olive oil, lemon juice, salt, and pepper to make the dressing.
    4. Pour the dressing over the salad and toss to coat.
    5. Serve the salmon fillets on top of the quinoa salad.
- **Where to get it:** Local fish market or grocery store.
- **Nutritional Value:** Salmon provides Vitamin D and omega-3 fatty acids, quinoa adds calcium and protein, while the lemon-herb dressing offers additional flavor and Vitamin C.

10. **Greek Yogurt and Berry Parfait with Almond Granola**

- **Ingredients:**
    - 1 cup Greek yogurt
    - 1/2 cup mixed berries (such as strawberries, blueberries, and raspberries)
    - 1/4 cup almond granola
    - Honey (optional)
- **Preparation:**
    1. In a glass or bowl, layer Greek yogurt, mixed berries, and almond granola.
    2. Drizzle with honey if desired.
    3. Repeat the layers until the glass or bowl is filled.
    4. Serve immediately as a nutritious breakfast or snack.
- **Where to get it:** Local grocery store.
- **Nutritional Value:** Greek yogurt provides Vitamin D and protein, berries add calcium and

antioxidants, while almond granola offers additional calcium and fiber.

11.Fatty Fish with Lemony Herbs

- **Ingredients:**
    - 2 fillets of fatty fish (such as salmon, mackerel, or trout)
    - 2 tablespoons olive oil
    - 2 cloves garlic, minced
    - 2 tablespoons fresh herbs (such as parsley, dill, or thyme), chopped
    - 1 lemon, sliced
    - Salt and pepper to taste
- **Preparation:**
    1. Preheat oven to 300°F (200°C).
    2. Place the fish fillets on a baking sheet lined with parchment paper.
    3. In a small bowl, mix together olive oil, minced garlic, chopped herbs, salt, and pepper.

4. Spread the herb mixture evenly over the fish fillets.
5. Place lemon slices on top of the fish.
6. Cook in the oven that has been preheated for 12-15 minutes, or until the fish is fully cooked and can be readily separated into flakes using a fork.
7. Serve hot, garnished with additional fresh herbs if desired.

12. Salmon Burgers with D-Fortified Mushrooms

- **Ingredients:**
    - 1 lb salmon fillet, skin removed
    - 1 cup mushrooms, finely chopped
    - 1/4 cup breadcrumbs
    - 1 egg, beaten
    - 2 tablespoons fresh parsley, chopped
    - 1 teaspoon lemon zest
    - Salt and pepper to taste
    - Olive oil for cooking
- **Preparation:**
    1. Using a food processor, chop the salmon until it is finely minced.
    2. Transfer the chopped salmon to a mixing bowl and add the chopped mushrooms, breadcrumbs, beaten egg, chopped parsley, lemon zest, salt, and

pepper. Mix until well combined.

3. Divide the mixture into 4 equal portions and shape each portion into a patty.
4. Heat olive oil in a pan over medium heat.
5. Cook the salmon burgers for 3-5 minutes on each side, or until golden brown and cooked through.
6. Serve the salmon burgers on whole grain buns with your favorite toppings, such as lettuce, tomato, and avocado.

13 Fortified Milk & OJ Breakfast Smoothie

- **Ingredients:**
    - 1 cup fortified milk (such as almond milk, soy milk, or cow's milk)
    - 1/2 cup orange juice (fortified with Vitamin D)
    - 1 ripe banana, peeled and sliced
    - 1/2 cup Greek yogurt
    - 1 tablespoon honey (optional)
    - Ice cubes
- **Preparation:**
    1. In a blender, combine the fortified milk, orange juice, sliced banana, Greek yogurt, and honey (if using).
    2. Put a few ice cubes into the mixer.
    3. Blend on high speed until smooth and creamy.

4. Taste the smoothie and adjust sweetness with more honey if desired.
5. Transfer the smoothie into cups and serve right away.
6. Optionally, garnish with a slice of orange or a sprinkle of chia seeds for added nutrition.

CHAPTER 3

Protein Power: Essential for Bone Health and Muscle Maintenance

1. **Grilled Chicken Breast with Quinoa and Steamed Broccoli**
   - **Ingredients:**
     - 2 chicken breasts
     - 1 cup cooked quinoa
     - 1 cup steamed broccoli florets
     - Olive oil
     - Salt and pepper
   - **Instructions:**
     1. Season chicken breasts with salt, pepper, and a drizzle of olive oil.
     2. Grill chicken until cooked through, about 7-8 minutes per side.
     3. Serve grilled chicken alongside cooked quinoa

and steamed broccoli for a protein-rich meal.

2. **Greek Yogurt Parfait with Mixed Berries and Almond Granola**
   - **Ingredients:**
     - 1 cup Greek yogurt
       One and half cup mixed berries (such as strawberries, blueberries, raspberries)
     - 1/4 cup almond granola
     - Honey (optional)
   - **Instructions:**
     1. In a glass or bowl, layer Greek yogurt, mixed berries, and almond granola.
     2. Repeat the layers until the glass or bowl is filled.
     3. Drizzle with honey if desired for added sweetness.

3. **Salmon and Avocado Salad with Lemon Vinaigrette**
   - **Ingredients:**
     - 4 oz grilled salmon
     - 1 ripe avocado, sliced
     - Mixed greens
     - Cherry tomatoes
     - Lemon vinaigrette (olive oil, lemon juice, Dijon mustard, salt, pepper)
   - **Instructions:**
     1. Arrange mixed greens, cherry tomatoes, and sliced avocado on a plate.
     2. Top with grilled salmon.
     3. Drizzle with lemon vinaigrette before serving.

4. **Turkey and Vegetable Stir-Fry with Brown Rice**
   - **Ingredients:**
       - 1 cup cooked brown rice
       - 8 oz turkey breast, thinly sliced
       - Mixed vegetables (bell peppers, broccoli, carrots)
       - Soy sauce
       - Garlic, minced
       - Olive oil
   - **Instructions:**
       1. Heat olive oil in a skillet or wok over medium-high heat.
       2. Add minced garlic and sliced turkey breast. Cook until turkey is browned.
       3. Add mixed vegetables and stir-fry until tender-crisp.
       4. Stir in cooked brown rice and soy sauce. Cook until heated through.

5. **Black Bean and Quinoa Salad with Cilantro-Lime Dressing**
   - **Ingredients:**
     - 1 cup cooked quinoa
     - 1 can black beans, rinsed and drained
     - Red bell pepper, diced
     - Red onion, diced
     - Fresh cilantro, chopped
     - Lime juice
     - Olive oil
     - Salt and pepper
   - **Instructions:**
     1. In a large bowl, combine cooked quinoa, black beans, diced bell pepper, and diced red onion.
     2. In a small bowl, whisk together lime juice, olive oil, chopped cilantro, salt, and pepper to make the dressing.
     3. Put the dressing over the salad and toss to combine.

6. **Egg and Spinach Breakfast Wrap**
   - **Ingredients:**
     - 2 large eggs
     - Handful of spinach leaves
     - Whole wheat wrap or tortilla
     - Shredded cheese (optional)
     - Salt and pepper
   - **Instructions:**
     1. Scramble eggs in a pan over medium heat until cooked through.
     2. Add spinach leaves to the pan and cook until wilted.
     3. Place scrambled eggs and spinach on a whole wheat wrap or tortilla.
     4. Optionally, sprinkle with shredded cheese before rolling up the wrap.

7. **Cottage Cheese and Fruit Bowl**
   - **Ingredients:**
     - 1/2 cup cottage cheese
     - Mixed fresh fruit (such as berries, sliced peaches, kiwi)
     - Honey (optional)
   - **Instructions:**
     1. Spoon cottage cheese into a bowl.
     2. Top with mixed fresh fruit.
     3. Drizzle with honey for added sweetness if desired.

8. **Tofu and Vegetable Stir-Fry with Rice Noodles**
   - **Ingredients:**
     - 8 oz firm tofu, cubed
     - Mixed vegetables (snap peas, carrots, bell peppers)
     - Rice noodles, cooked
     - Soy sauce
     - Garlic, minced
     - Ginger, grated
     - Sesame oil

- **Instructions:**
    1. 1. Warm up sesame oil in a skillet or wok on medium-high heat.
    2. Add minced garlic and grated ginger, followed by cubed tofu. Cook until tofu is golden brown.
    3. Add mixed vegetables and stir-fry until tender-crisp.
    4. Stir in cooked rice noodles and soy sauce.
    5. Cook until it heated well.

9. Chickpea and Spinach Curry with Brown Rice

Ingredients: •

1 can chickpeas, washed and drained • Fresh spinach leaves

- Onion, diced
- Garlic, minced
- Curry powder
- Coconut milk
- Prepared brown rice

Directions:
1. Cook chopped onion and minced garlic in a pot until they become soft.
2. Add curry powder and simmer till aromatic.
3. Stir in chickpeas, fresh spinach leaves, and coconut milk. Simmer until spinach wilts.
4. Serve curry over cooked brown rice.

10. Peanut Butter Banana Smoothie •
Ingredients:
1 ripe banana
• 2 tablespoons peanut butter
• 1 cup milk (dairy or plant-based)
• Honey or maple syrup (optional)
• Ice cubes

Instructions:
1. Combine banana, peanut butter, milk, and honey or maple syrup (if using) in a blender.
2. Add a handful of ice cubes.
3. Blend until smooth and creamy.
4. Pour into glasses and serve immediately.

Lean Chicken Stir-Fry •
Ingredients:
2 boneless, skinless chicken breasts, thinly sliced
2 cups mixed veggies (such as bell peppers, broccoli, carrots, snap peas)
• 2 cloves garlic, minced
• 2 tablespoons soy sauce
• 1 tablespoon sesame oil
• 1 tablespoon cornstarch
• 2 teaspoons olive oil
• Salt and pepper to taste
Instructions:
1. In a small bowl, mix soy sauce, sesame oil, and cornstarch to form the sauce. Set aside.
2. Heat olive oil in a large skillet or wok over medium-high heat.
3. Add minced garlic and sliced chicken breasts to the skillet. Cook until chicken is no longer pink.
4. Add mixed vegetables to the skillet and stir-fry until tender-crisp.
5. Pour the sauce over the chicken and

vegetables. Stir until the sauce thickens and coats everything evenly.
6. Season with salt and pepper to taste.
7. Serve the stir-fry hot over prepared rice or noodles.

2. Poached Fish with Citrus Sauce

Ingredients:
4 fish fillets (such as tilapia, cod, or sole)
• 2 cups fish or vegetable broth
• 1 orange, juiced
1 lemon, juiced
2 cloves garlic, minced
• 1 tablespoon olive oil
• Salt and pepper to taste

Instructions:
1. In a big skillet or shallow pan, bring fish or vegetable broth to a simmer.
2. Add minced garlic, orange juice, lemon juice, and olive oil to the simmering soup.
3. Season fish fillets with salt and pepper, then gently add them to the simmering liquid.

4. Poach fish for 5-7 minutes, or until it is opaque and flakes readily with a fork.
5. Remove fish from the broth and transfer to serving plates.
6. Spoon citrus sauce over the poached fish before serving.
7. Garnish with fresh herbs, if preferred.

Lentil Soup with Sausage

Ingredients:
1 cup dried lentils, rinsed and drained
• 4 cups chicken or vegetable broth
• 2 Italian sausages, sliced
• 1 onion, diced
• 2 carrots, diced
• 2 celery stalks, diced
• 2 cloves garlic, minced
• 1 can diced tomatoes
• 1 teaspoon dried thyme
• Salt and pepper to taste
• Olive oil

Instructions:

1. Heat olive oil in a big pot over medium heat. Add diced onion, carrots, celery, and minced garlic. Cook until vegetables are softened.
2. Add sliced Italian sausages to the pot and simmer until browned.
3. Stir in dried lentils, chopped tomatoes, dried thyme, and chicken or vegetable broth. Bring to a boil.
4. Reduce heat to medium and simmer the soup, covered, for 20-25 minutes, or until lentils are cooked.
5. Season with salt and pepper to taste.
6. Serve the lentil soup hot, garnished with fresh herbs if preferred.

CHAPTER 4

Veggies for Vibrant Bones: The Importance of Fruits & Vegetables

Rainbow Veggie and Fruit Salad with Citrus Dressing

Ingredients:

♣ 2 cups mixed salad greens (such as spinach, kale, arugula)

♣ 1 cup mixed colorful veggies (such as bell peppers, cherry tomatoes, cucumber, shredded carrots)

♣ 1 cup assorted fresh fruits (such as strawberries, oranges, kiwi, blueberries)

♣ one-quarter cup of sliced almonds or walnuts (optional)

Instructions:

- In a large bowl, toss together mixed salad greens, colorful vegetables, and fresh fruits.
- If using, sprinkle sliced almonds or walnuts over the salad for added crunch.
- In a small bowl, whisk together olive oil, fresh lemon juice, honey or maple syrup, salt, and pepper to make the citrus dressing.
- Drizzle the citrus dressing over the salad and toss gently to coat everything evenly.
- Serve the rainbow veggie and fruit salad as a refreshing and nutritious side dish or light meal.

Roasted Vegetable Medley with Balsamic Glaze

Ingredients:

2 cups mixed veggies (such as bell peppers, zucchini, eggplant, cherry tomatoes)
♣ 2 tablespoons olive oil
♣ Salt and pepper to taste
♣ Balsamic glaze (store-bought or homemade)

Instructions:
Heat the oven to 400°F (200°C).
 Cut the vegetables into bite-sized pieces and lay them on a baking sheet.
♣Spray olive oil over the vegetables and season with salt and pepper.
♣ Mix the crops to coat them evenly with oil and seasoning.
♣ Roast in the hot oven for 20-25 minutes, or until the vegetables are soft and gently browned.
♣ Pour with honey sauce before dishing. ☐
Fruit and Veggie Smoothie Bowl

Ingredients:

1 ripe banana

♣ 1/2 cup mixed berries (such as strawberries, blueberries, raspberries)

♣ 1/2 cup of various greens (such as spinach, kale)

♣ 1/4 cup diced mango ♣ 1/4 cup diced cucumber

 1/4 cup almond milk

Toppings: sliced kiwi, granola, shredded coconut, chia seeds

Instructions:

In a blender, add banana, mixed berries, mixed greens, diced mango, diced cucumber, and almond milk.

♣ Blend until smooth and creamy, adding more almond milk if required to reach desired consistency.

♣ Pour the smoothie into a bowl.

 Top with sliced kiwi, granola, shredded coconut, and chia seeds.

♣ Enjoy this colorful and nutrient-packed smoothie bowl for breakfast or as a refreshing snack.

Stuffed Bell Peppers with Quinoa and Black
Beans

Ingredients:
4 bell peppers (any color), halved and
seeded
- 1 cup cooked quinoa
- 1 cup black beans, cooked
- 1 cup diced tomatoes
- 1/2 cup corn kernels
- 1/4 cup chopped cilantro
- 1 teaspoon cumin
- 1/2 teaspoon chili powder
- Salt and pepper to taste
- Sliced cheese (optional)

- **Instructions:**
  Prepare the oven to 375°F (190°C).
  In a large bowl, mix together cooked
  quinoa, black beans, diced tomatoes,
  corn kernels, chopped cilantro, cumin,
  chili powder, salt, and pepper.

Stuff the half bell peppers with the quinoa and black bean mixture.

♣Place the stuffed bell peppers on a baking dish.

♣If preferred, put shredded cheese on top of the stuffed bell peppers.

♣Bake in the preheated oven for 25-30 minutes, or until the peppers are soft and the filling is heated through.

♣ Serve the stuffed bell peppers hot, topped with more chopped cilantro if desired.

Rainbow Veggie Skewers with Lemon-Herb Marinade

- **Ingredients:**
  Assorted colorful veggies (such as cherry tomatoes, bell peppers, zucchini, red onion, mushrooms)
- Wooden skewers, soaked in water
  2 tablespoons olive oil
  Juice of 1 lemon
  1-2 cloves garlic, minced ♣
  1 teaspoon dried herbs (such as thyme,

rosemary, oregano) Salt and pepper to
taste

Instructions:
Set the grill to medium-high heat.
Thread assorted colorful vegetables onto
the moistened wooden skewers,
alternating colors.
 In a small bowl, whisk together olive oil,
lemon juice, minced garlic, dried herbs,
salt, and pepper to form the marinade.
♣Brush the veggie skewers with the
lemon-herb marinade.
♣Grill the skewers for 8-10 minutes,
rotating regularly, until the vegetables are
cooked and lightly browned.
♣Offer the rainbow veggie skewers hot as
a vibrant and healthful side dish.

Mixed Fruit Salad with Honey-Lime Dressing

Ingredients:

- Assorted fresh fruits (such as strawberries, pineapple, mango, grapes, kiwi, oranges)
- 2 tablespoons honey
- Juice of 1 lime
- Fresh mint leaves for garnish

Instructions:

- Cut the assorted fresh fruits into bite-sized pieces and place them in a large bowl.
- In a small bowl, whisk together honey and lime juice to make the dressing.
- Pour the honey-lime dressing over the mixed fruit salad and toss gently to coat.
- Garnish with fresh mint leaves before serving.
- Enjoy this colorful and refreshing fruit salad as a healthy dessert or snack option.

CHAPTER 6

30-Breakfast Recipes To support a healthy bone for your family or yourself

Avocado Toast with Poached Egg:

Ingredients:

Avocado, whole grain bread, eggs, salt, pepper, optional toppings (e.g., cherry tomatoes, feta cheese, red pepper flakes).

Instructions: Toast bread, mash avocado onto toast, poach egg, place egg on top of avocado, season with salt and pepper, add optional toppings if desired.

Nutritional values (per serving): Calories: 300, Protein: 12g, Fat: 18g, Carbohydrates: 25g, Fiber: 7g.

Greek Yogurt Parfait with Granola and Fresh Fruit:

Ingredients: Greek yogurt, granola, fresh fruit (e.g., berries, banana, kiwi), honey or maple syrup (optional).

Instructions: Layer Greek yogurt, granola, and fresh fruit in a glass or bowl, drizzle with honey or maple syrup if desired.

Nutritional values (per serving): Calories: 300, Protein: 15g, Fat: 8g, Carbohydrates: 45g, Fiber: 6g.

Veggie Omelette with Cheese:

Ingredients: Eggs, bell peppers, onions, tomatoes, spinach, cheese (e.g., cheddar, feta), salt, pepper, cooking oil.

Instructions: Beat eggs, chop vegetables, sauté vegetables in oil, pour beaten eggs over vegetables, cook until set, sprinkle with cheese, fold omelette in half, season with salt and pepper.

Nutritional values (per serving): Calories: 250, Protein: 18g, Fat: 16g, Carbohydrates: 8g, Fiber: 3g.

Banana Walnut Muffins:

Ingredients: All-purpose flour, ripe bananas, walnuts, eggs, butter, sugar, baking powder, salt, vanilla extract.

Instructions: Mash bananas, mix wet ingredients, mix dry ingredients, combine wet and dry ingredients, fold in walnuts, pour into muffin tin, bake.

Nutritional values (per serving): Calories: 220, Protein: 4g, Fat: 10g, Carbohydrates: 30g, Fiber: 2g.

Breakfast Burrito with Sausage, Egg, and Cheese:

Ingredients: Tortillas, breakfast sausage, eggs, cheese, bell peppers, onions, salsa (optional), salt, pepper.

Instructions: Cook sausage, scramble eggs, assemble burritos with sausage, eggs, cheese, vegetables, and salsa, wrap burritos, heat in skillet until cheese melts.

Nutritional values (per serving): Calories: 400, Protein: 18g, Fat: 25g, Carbohydrates: 28g, Fiber: 3g.

Blueberry Almond Smoothie Bowl:

Ingredients: Frozen blueberries, almond milk, almond butter, banana, spinach, toppings (e.g., sliced almonds, chia seeds, granola, fresh blueberries).

Instructions: Blend blueberries, almond milk, almond butter, banana, and spinach until smooth, pour into bowl, add toppings.

Nutritional values (per serving): Calories: 350, Protein: 8g, Fat: 15g, Carbohydrates: 50g, Fiber: 12g.

Smoked Salmon and Cream Cheese Bagel:

Ingredients: Bagels, smoked salmon, cream cheese, red onion, capers, lemon, salt, pepper.

Instructions: Toast bagels, spread cream cheese on each half, top with smoked salmon, thinly sliced red onion, capers, a squeeze of lemon juice, and season with salt and pepper.

Nutritional values (per serving): Calories: 380, Protein: 20g, Fat: 12g, Carbohydrates: 45g, Fiber: 3g.

Quinoa Breakfast Bowl with Roasted Veggies:

Ingredients: Quinoa, bell peppers, zucchini, cherry tomatoes, olive oil, salt, pepper, eggs, avocado (optional).

Instructions: Cook quinoa, roast chopped vegetables tossed in olive oil, season with salt and pepper, fry eggs, assemble bowls with quinoa, roasted veggies, and fried eggs, top with sliced avocado if desired.

Nutritional values

Calories: 420, Protein: 15g, Fat: 18g, Carbohydrates: 52g, Fiber: 9g.

Apple Cinnamon Overnight French Toast Bake:

Ingredients: Bread slices, apples, eggs, milk, cinnamon, vanilla extract, maple syrup.

Instructions: Arrange bread slices in a baking dish, layer with sliced apples, whisk together eggs, milk, cinnamon, and vanilla extract, pour mixture over bread and apples, cover and refrigerate overnight, bake in the morning, serve with maple syrup.

Nutritional values Calories: 320, Protein: 12g, Fat: 8g, Carbohydrates: 50g, Fiber: 6g.

Spinach and Mushroom Breakfast Quesadilla:

Ingredients: Tortillas, spinach, mushrooms, eggs, cheese (e.g., Monterey Jack), salt, pepper, cooking oil.

Instructions: Sauté spinach and mushrooms, scramble eggs, assemble quesadillas with sautéed veggies, scrambled eggs, and cheese between tortillas, cook in a skillet until golden and cheese is melted.

Nutritional values (per serving): Calories: 340, Protein: 15g, Fat: 18g, Carbohydrates: 30g, Fiber: 5g.

Chia Seed Pudding with Mixed Berries:

Ingredients: Chia seeds, almond milk, honey or maple syrup, mixed berries (e.g., strawberries, blueberries, raspberries).

Instructions: Mix chia seeds, almond milk, and sweetener, refrigerate overnight, serve with mixed berries on top.

Nutritional values (per serving): Calories: 220, Protein: 5g, Fat: 10g, Carbohydrates: 30g, Fiber: 10g.

Breakfast Tacos with Black Beans and Avocado:

Ingredients: Corn tortillas, black beans, eggs, avocado, salsa, cilantro, lime, salt, pepper.

Instructions: Warm tortillas, scramble eggs, heat black beans, assemble tacos with eggs, black beans, sliced avocado, salsa, and garnish with chopped cilantro and a squeeze of lime juice, season with salt and pepper.

Nutritional values (per serving): Calories: 350, Protein: 15g, Fat: 15g, Carbohydrates: 40g, Fiber: 12g.

Peanut Butter Banana Overnight Oats:

Ingredients: Rolled oats, almond milk, peanut butter, banana, honey or maple syrup, cinnamon (optional).

Instructions: Mix oats, almond milk, peanut butter, mashed banana, sweetener, and cinnamon, refrigerate overnight, serve chilled.

Nutritional values (per serving): Calories: 380, Protein: 10g, Fat: 15g, Carbohydrates: 50g, Fiber: 8g.

Coconut Mango Smoothie:

Ingredients: Frozen mango chunks, coconut milk, Greek yogurt, honey or agave syrup, shredded coconut (optional).

Instructions: Blend mango chunks, coconut milk, Greek yogurt, and sweetener until smooth, garnish with shredded coconut if desired.

Nutritional values (per serving): Calories: 280, Protein: 10g, Fat: 10g, Carbohydrates: 40g, Fiber: 5g.

Bacon, Egg, and Cheese Breakfast Sandwich:

Ingredients: English muffins, bacon, eggs, cheese (e.g., American, cheddar), butter, salt, pepper.

Instructions: Cook bacon until crispy, fry eggs, toast English muffins, assemble sandwiches with bacon, eggs, cheese, buttered English muffins, season with salt and pepper.

Nutritional values (per serving): Calories: 450, Protein: 20g, Fat: 25g, Carbohydrates: 30g, Fiber: 2g.

Sweet Potato Hash with Fried Eggs:

Ingredients: Sweet potatoes, bell peppers, onions, garlic, eggs, cooking oil, salt, pepper, paprika (optional).

Instructions: Dice sweet potatoes and vegetables, sauté in oil until tender, fry eggs, serve eggs over sweet potato hash, season with salt, pepper, and paprika if desired.

Nutritional values (per serving): Calories: 320, Protein: 12g, Fat: 15g, Carbohydrates: 35g, Fiber: 6g.

Raspberry Chocolate Chip Pancakes:

Ingredients: Pancake mix, milk, eggs, raspberries, chocolate chips, butter or cooking spray.

Instructions: Prepare pancake batter according to package instructions, fold in raspberries and chocolate chips, cook pancakes on a griddle or skillet with butter or cooking spray until golden brown on both sides.

Nutritional values (per serving): Calories: 350, Protein: 8g, Fat: 12g, Carbohydrates: 50g, Fiber: 4g.

Breakfast Casserole with Hash Browns and Sausage:

Ingredients: Hash browns, breakfast sausage, eggs, milk, cheese, bell peppers, onions, salt, pepper.

Instructions: Cook breakfast sausage, layer hash browns, cooked sausage, chopped vegetables, and cheese in a baking dish, whisk together eggs, milk, salt, and pepper, pour over the layers, bake until set and golden brown.

Nutritional values (per serving): Calories: 420, Protein: 18g, Fat: 25g, Carbohydrates: 30g, Fiber: 3g.

Sourdough Breakfast Pizza with Bacon and Eggs:

Ingredients: Sourdough bread, bacon, eggs, cheese (e.g., mozzarella, cheddar), tomatoes, spinach, olive oil, salt, pepper.

Instructions: Toast sourdough bread, cook bacon until crispy, fry eggs, assemble pizzas with toasted sourdough as the base, topped with bacon, eggs, cheese, tomatoes, and spinach, drizzle with olive oil, season with salt and pepper, bake until cheese melts.

Nutritional values (per serving): Calories: 380, Protein: 20g, Fat: 18g, Carbohydrates: 30g, Fiber: 3g.

Veggie Breakfast Wrap with Hummus:

Ingredients: Whole wheat wraps, hummus, scrambled eggs, bell peppers, onions, spinach, feta cheese, salt, pepper.

Instructions: Spread hummus on wraps, fill with scrambled eggs, sautéed vegetables, and crumbled feta cheese, season with salt and pepper, wrap tightly.

Nutritional values (per serving): Calories: 320, Protein: 15g, Fat: 12g, Carbohydrates: 40g, Fiber: 7g.

Pumpkin Spice Waffles:

Ingredients: Waffle mix, pumpkin puree, milk, eggs, pumpkin pie spice, maple syrup, whipped cream (optional).

Instructions: Mix waffle batter with pumpkin puree, milk, eggs, and pumpkin pie spice, cook in waffle iron until golden brown, and serve with maple syrup and whipped cream if desired.

Nutritional values (per serving): Calories: 300, Protein: 8g, Fat: 10g, Carbohydrates: 45g, Fiber: 3g.

CHAPTER 7

Lunchtime: Easy and Nutritious Options for Seniors

1. **Vegetable and Bean Soup:**
   - **Ingredients:** Mixed vegetables (such as carrots, celery, onions, spinach), beans (such as kidney beans, chickpeas), low-sodium vegetable broth, garlic, herbs (such as thyme, rosemary), olive oil, salt, pepper.
   - **Instructions:** Sauté mixed vegetables and garlic in olive oil, add beans, vegetable broth, and herbs.
   - Simmer until vegetables are done. Serve hot.
2. **Grilled Chicken Wrap:**
   - **Ingredients:** Grilled chicken breast strips, whole wheat tortilla, lettuce, tomato, avocado, Greek yogurt or hummus (as spread), salt, pepper.
   - **Instructions**: Spread Greek yogurt or hummus on a whole wheat tortilla, add grilled chicken breast strips,

lettuce, tomato, and avocado. Roll up tightly and slice.

3. **Quinoa and Vegetable Stir-Fry:**
    - **Ingredients:** Quinoa, mixed vegetables (such as bell peppers, broccoli, snap peas), tofu or cooked chicken strips, soy sauce, garlic, ginger, sesame oil, green onions, salt, pepper.
    - **Instructions:** Cook quinoa according to package instructions. Sauté mixed vegetables, tofu or chicken strips in sesame oil with garlic, ginger, soy sauce, salt, and pepper. Serve over cooked quinoa, garnish with green onions.

4. **Greek Yogurt Parfait:**
    - Ingredients: Greek yogurt, mixed berries (such as strawberries, blueberries, raspberries), granola, honey or maple syrup, nuts (such as almonds, walnuts).
    - Instructions: Layer Greek yogurt with mixed berries, granola, and nuts in a

bowl or glass. Drizzle with honey or maple syrup for sweetness.

5. **Tuna Salad Sandwich:**
   - **Ingredients:** Canned tuna, whole grain bread, lettuce, tomato, red onion, Greek yogurt (as a healthier alternative to mayo), mustard, salt, pepper.
   - **Instructions:** Mix canned tuna with Greek yogurt, mustard, salt, and pepper. Spread on whole grain bread and top with lettuce, tomato, and red onion slices.

some convenient lunch options for people at work who may not have time to cook, along with stores where they can purchase them immediately.

1. **Pre-made Salad Kits from Grocery Stores:**
   - **Stores:** Whole Foods, Trader Joe's, Kroger, Walmart.
   - **Nutritional Value:** Varies depending on the kit, but typically includes a mix of greens, vegetables, protein (such as grilled chicken or tofu), nuts or seeds, and dressing. Look for options with lean protein and plenty of vegetables for a balanced meal.
2. **Ready-to-Eat Sushi Rolls:**
   - **Stores:** Wegmans, Safeway, Target, Costco.
   - **Nutritional Value:** Sushi rolls typically provide protein from fish or tofu, carbohydrates from rice, and some vegetables. Opt for rolls with

lean fish like tuna or salmon and brown rice for added fiber.

3. **Pre-packaged Wraps or Sandwiches:**
   - **Stores:** Starbucks, Panera Bread, Subway, convenience stores.
   - **Nutritional Value:** Look for wraps or sandwiches with whole grain bread or wraps, lean protein (such as turkey or grilled chicken), plenty of vegetables, and minimal added sauces or dressings.
   - Check nutrition labels for calorie, protein, and sodium content.

4. **Greek Yogurt with Granola and Fruit:**
   - **Stores:** Target, CVS, gas stations, convenience stores.
   - **Nutritional Value:** Greek yogurt provides protein and calcium, while granola and fruit add fiber and vitamins. Look for plain Greek yogurt to avoid added sugars, and choose granola with whole grains and minimal added sugars.

5. **Pre-packaged Salad Bowls:**
   - **Stores:** Costco, Trader Joe's, Whole Foods, convenience stores.
   - **Nutritional Value:** These typically include a mix of greens, vegetables, protein (such as grilled chicken or hard-boiled eggs), cheese, nuts or seeds, and dressing. Look for options with a variety of colorful vegetables and lean protein sources.
6. **Protein Bars or Meal Replacement Bars:**
   - **Stores:** GNC, Walgreens, CVS, gas stations, convenience stores.
   - **Nutritional Value:** Choose bars with a balance of protein, carbohydrates, and healthy fats. Look for options with at least 10 grams of protein and less than 10 grams of added sugars. Check labels for fiber content and overall calorie count.

7. **Pre-cut Fruit and Veggie Trays:**
   - Stores: Costco, Walmart, Kroger, Whole Foods, convenience stores.
   - Nutritional Value: These trays typically include a variety of fresh fruits and vegetables, providing vitamins, minerals, and fiber. Pair with hummus or Greek yogurt dip for added protein and flavor.

8. **Rotisserie Chicken with Ready-to-Eat Sides:**
   - **Stores:** Costco, Sam's Club, Whole Foods, grocery stores with deli sections.
   - **Nutritional Value:** Rotisserie chicken provides protein and can be paired with ready-to-eat sides like pre-cut vegetables, salad kits, or pre-cooked grains for a balanced meal. Opt for skinless chicken and choose sides with minimal added sauces or dressings.

9. **Frozen Meals:**
   - **Stores:** Target, Walmart, Trader Joe's, Whole Foods, convenience stores.
   - **Nutritional Value:** Look for frozen meals with whole food ingredients, balanced macronutrients (protein, carbohydrates, and fats), and limited added sugars and sodium. Choose options with lean protein sources, plenty of vegetables, and whole grains.

10. **Protein Smoothies or Shakes:**
    - **Stores:** Smoothie shops (e.g., Smoothie King, Jamba Juice), convenience stores, grocery stores.
    - **Nutritional Value:** Protein smoothies or shakes can provide a quick and portable meal option. Look for options made with protein powder, fruits, vegetables, and healthy fats (such as nut butter or avocado). Be mindful of added sugars and portion sizes.

11. **Soup Cups or Instant Noodle Cups:**

- **Stores:** Grocery stores, convenience stores, Asian markets.
- **Nutritional Value:** Choose soups or noodle cups with broth-based soups, lean protein (such as chicken or tofu), plenty of vegetables, and whole grain noodles.
- Look for options with lower sodium content and avoid those with excessive added MSG or preservatives.

PLEASE MAKE SURE TO BE CHECKING THE LAELS BEFORE BUYING

12. **Pre-packaged Hummus with Veggie Sticks and Whole Grain Crackers:**

- **Stores:** Target, Walmart, Costco, grocery stores, convenience stores.
- **Nutritional Value:** Hummus provides plant-based protein and healthy fats, while veggie sticks (such as carrots, bell peppers, and cucumber slices) and whole grain crackers offer fiber and additional nutrients.
- Choose hummus without added oils or preservatives for a healthier option.

13. **Nut Butter Sandwich on Whole Grain Bread:**

- **Stores:** Grocery stores, convenience stores, gas stations.
- **Nutritional Value:** Spread natural nut butter (such as almond or peanut butter) on whole-grain bread for a quick and satisfying

meal. Pair with sliced banana or apple for added sweetness and fiber. Look for bread with minimal added sugars and artificial ingredients.

And hey, if you ever need more recipes or cooking tips, you know where to find me! Check my Author. Share with your friend to select the solution to what they are going through.

CHAPTER 8

Dinnertime Delectables: Satisfying and Bone-Building Main Courses

1.Vegetable and Chickpea Curry:

- **Ingredients:** Chickpeas, mixed vegetables (such as bell peppers, cauliflower, peas), coconut milk, curry paste, onion, garlic, ginger, olive oil, salt, pepper, cilantro (for garnish).
- **Instructions:** Sauté onion, garlic, and ginger in olive oil until fragrant. Add curry paste and cook for a minute.
- Stir in mixed vegetables, chickpeas, and coconut milk. Simmer until vegetables are tender.
- Garnish with cilantro before serving.
- **Nutritional values (per serving):**

- Calories: 320
- Protein: 12g
- Fat: 10g
- Carbohydrates: 45g
- Fiber: 10g

2. Mushroom and Spinach Risotto:

- **Ingredients:** Arborio rice, mushrooms (such as cremini or shiitake), baby spinach, vegetable broth, onion, garlic, white wine, Parmesan cheese, olive oil, salt, pepper.
- **Instructions:** Sauté onion and garlic in olive oil until softened. Add mushrooms and cook until browned. Stir in Arborio rice and cook for a minute. Add white wine and cook until absorbed. Gradually add vegetable broth, stirring frequently, until rice is creamy. Stir in baby spinach and Parmesan cheese before serving.
- **Nutritional values (per serving):**
    - Calories: 380

- Protein: 10g
- Fat: 8g
- Carbohydrates: 60g
- Fiber: 5g

3.Teriyaki Beef and Broccoli Stir-Fry:

- Ingredients: Beef sirloin strips, broccoli florets, soy sauce, garlic, ginger, honey, cornstarch, sesame oil, green onions, sesame seeds, rice.
- Instructions: Marinate beef sirloin strips in a mixture of soy sauce, minced garlic, minced ginger, honey, and cornstarch. Stir-fry beef until browned. Add broccoli and cook until tender-crisp. Stir in a mixture of soy sauce and cornstarch until thickened. Serve over cooked rice and garnish with green onions and sesame seeds.
- Nutritional values (per serving):
  - Calories: 420
  - Protein: 25g
  - Fat: 15g

- Carbohydrates: 45g
- Fiber: 6g

8. **Lemon Herb Roasted Chicken:**
   - Ingredients: Chicken thighs or breasts, lemon juice, olive oil, garlic, rosemary, thyme, salt, pepper, potatoes, carrots.
   - Instructions: Marinate chicken in a mixture of lemon juice, olive oil, minced garlic, chopped rosemary, chopped thyme, salt, and pepper. Roast chicken with potatoes and carrots until golden brown and cooked through.
   - Nutritional values (per serving):
     - Calories: 380
     - Protein: 30g
     - Fat: 20g
     - Carbohydrates: 20g
     - Fiber: 3g

9. **Shrimp and Vegetable Stir-Fry:**
   - Ingredients: Shrimp, mixed vegetables (such as bell peppers, snap peas, carrots), soy sauce, garlic, ginger, sesame oil, cornstarch, green onions, rice.
   - Instructions: Marinate shrimp in a mixture of soy sauce, minced garlic, minced ginger, and cornstarch. Stir-fry shrimp and mixed vegetables in sesame oil until cooked through. Dish over cooked rice and garnish with sliced green onion slices.
   - Nutritional values (per serving):
     - Calories: 300
     - Protein: 25g
     - Fat: 10g
     - Carbohydrates: 35g
     - Fiber: 5g

10.   **Eggplant Parmesan:**

- Ingredients: Eggplant, breadcrumbs, grated Parmesan cheese, marinara sauce, mozzarella cheese, olive oil, Italian seasoning, salt, pepper.
- Instructions: Slice eggplant and coat in breadcrumbs mixed with grated Parmesan cheese, Italian seasoning, salt, and pepper. Bake until golden brown. Layer eggplant slices with marinara sauce and mozzarella cheese. Bake until cheese is bubbling and browned.
- Nutritional values (per serving):
  - Calories: 320
  - Protein: 15g
  - Fat: 12g
  - Carbohydrates: 40g
  - Fiber: 8g

13. **Vegetarian Butternut Squash and Black Bean Enchiladas:**

- Ingredients: Butternut squash, black beans, corn tortillas, enchilada sauce, onion, garlic, cumin, chili powder, cilantro, lime, cheese (optional).
- Instructions: Roast butternut squash until tender. Sauté onion and garlic, then mix with mashed black beans, roasted squash, cumin, chili powder, and chopped cilantro. Fill corn tortillas with the mixture, roll up, and place in a baking dish. Pour enchilada sauce over the top and bake until bubbly. Serve with lime wedges.
- Nutritional values (per serving):
    - Calories: 350
    - Protein: 12g
    - Fat: 8g
    - Carbohydrates: 60g
    - Fiber: 12g

14. **Honey Garlic Glazed Salmon with Roasted Vegetables:**
- Ingredients: Salmon fillets, honey, garlic, soy sauce, olive oil, mixed vegetables (such as carrots, Brussels sprouts, potatoes), salt, pepper.
- Instructions: Mix honey, minced garlic, and soy sauce to make the glaze. Brush over salmon fillets and bake until cooked through. Toss mixed vegetables with olive oil, salt, and pepper, then roast until tender. Serve salmon with roasted vegetables.
- Nutritional values (per serving):
  - Calories: 400
  - Protein: 30g
  - Fat: 18g
  - Carbohydrates: 30g
  - Fiber: 8g

15. **Turkey and Vegetable Meatballs with Whole Wheat Pasta:**

- Ingredients: Ground turkey, mixed vegetables (such as bell peppers, zucchini, onions), whole wheat pasta, marinara sauce, Parmesan cheese, egg, breadcrumbs, garlic, Italian seasoning, salt, pepper.
- Instructions: Mix ground turkey with chopped vegetables, egg, breadcrumbs, minced garlic, Italian seasoning, salt, and pepper. Form into meatballs and bake until cooked through. Serve over cooked whole wheat pasta with marinara sauce and grated Parmesan cheese.
- Nutritional values (per serving):
    - Calories: 380
    - Protein: 25g
    - Fat: 12g
    - Carbohydrates: 45g
    - Fiber: 10g

16. **Sesame Ginger Tofu Stir-Fry:**
- Ingredients: Firm tofu, mixed vegetables (such as bell peppers, snap peas, broccoli), soy sauce, garlic, ginger, sesame oil, cornstarch, green onions, sesame seeds, rice.
- Instructions: Press tofu to remove excess moisture, then cut into cubes and toss with cornstarch. Stir-fry tofu until golden brown, then set aside. Stir-fry mixed vegetables in sesame oil with minced garlic and ginger until tender-crisp. Add tofu back to the pan, along with soy sauce, and cook until heated through. Serve over cooked rice, garnished with sliced green onions and sesame seeds.

- Nutritional values (per serving):
  - Calories: 320
  - Protein: 20g
  - Fat: 15g
  - Carbohydrates: 30g
  - Fiber: 6g

17. **Mediterranean Stuffed Bell Peppers:**

  - Ingredients: Bell peppers, quinoa, chickpeas, cherry tomatoes, cucumber, red onion, Kalamata olives, feta cheese, olive oil, lemon juice, garlic, oregano, salt, and pepper.

  - Instructions: Cook quinoa according to package instructions. Mix cooked quinoa with chickpeas, halved cherry tomatoes, diced cucumber, chopped red onion, sliced Kalamata olives, crumbled feta cheese, minced garlic, olive oil, lemon juice, oregano, salt, and pepper. Stuff mixture into halved bell peppers and bake until peppers are tender.

- Nutritional values (per serving):
  - Calories: 340
  - Protein: 15g
  - Fat: 10g
  - Carbohydrates: 45g
  - Fiber: 10g

18. **Honey Mustard Glazed Pork Chops with Roasted Sweet Potatoes:**

- Ingredients: Pork chops, sweet potatoes, honey, Dijon mustard, olive oil, garlic powder, thyme, salt, and pepper.
- **Instructions: Mix honey, Dijon mustard, olive oil, garlic powder, minced thyme, salt, and pepper to make the glaze. Brush over pork chops and bake until cooked through. Toss sweet potato wedges with olive oil, salt, and pepper, then roast until tender. Serve pork chops with roasted sweet potatoes.**
- **Nutritional values (per serving):**
  - **Calories: 420**

- **Protein: 30g**
- **Fat: 18g**
- **Carbohydrates: 35g**
- Fiber: 6g

CHAPTER 9

Sweet Endings: Healthy and Delicious Desserts for Seniors

1. **Baked Apples with Cinnamon:**
   - **Ingredients:** Apples, cinnamon, honey (optional), chopped nuts (optional).
   - Instructions:
     1. Preheat the oven to 375°F (190°C).
     2. Core the apples and set them in a baking dish.
     3. Sprinkle cinnamon over the apples and drizzle with honey if desired.

4. Bake for 20-25 minutes or until the apples are tender.
5. Serve warm, optionally topped with chopped nuts.

2. **Yogurt Parfaits with Fruit & Granola:**
   - **Ingredients:**

   Greek yogurt, fresh mixed berries (such as strawberries, blueberries, raspberries), granola, honey (optional).

   - **Instructions:**
     1. In serving mug or bowls, layer Greek yogurt, fresh mixed berries, and granola.
     2. Repeat the layers until the glass or bowl is filled.
     3. Drizzle with honey if desired.
     4. Serve immediately or refrigerate until ready to serve.

3. **Chia Seed Pudding with Berries:**
    - Ingredients: Chia seeds, milk (dairy or plant-based), honey or maple syrup, vanilla extract, mixed berries (such as strawberries, blackberries, raspberries).
    - Instructions:
        1. In a bowl, mix chia seeds, milk, honey or maple syrup, and vanilla extract.
        2. Mixture it for 5 minutes, then stir again to prevent clumping.
        3. Cover the bowl and refrigerate for at least 2 hours or overnight until the mixture thickens and becomes pudding-like.
        4. Serve the chia seed pudding topped with mixed berries.

4. **Frozen Banana "Ice Cream" with Peanut Butter:**
  - **Ingredients:**
  - Ripe bananas, peanut butter (or almond butter), cocoa powder (optional), chopped nuts (optional).
  - Instructions:
    1. Peel ripe bananas and slice them into coins.
    2. Place the banana slices in a single layer on a baking sheet lined with parchment paper and freeze until firm, about 2 hours.
    3. Once frozen, transfer the banana slices to a food processor or blender.
    4. Add a spoonful of peanut butter (or almond butter) and cocoa powder if desired.
    5. Blend until smooth and creamy, scraping down the sides as needed.

6. Serve immediately as soft-serve "ice cream" or freeze for a firmer texture.
7. Optional: Sprinkle chopped nuts on top before serving for added crunch.

5. **Fruit Salad with Honey-Lime Dressing:**
   - Ingredients: Assorted fruits (such as strawberries, kiwi, pineapple, grapes, oranges), honey, lime juice, fresh mint leaves (optional).
   - Instructions:
     1. Wash, peel, and chop the assorted fruits into bite-sized pieces.
     2. In a small bowl, whisk together honey and lime juice to make the dressing.
     3. Drizzle the honey-lime dressing over the chopped fruits and gently toss to coat.
     4. Garnish with fresh mint leaves if desired.

5. Serve immediately or chill in the refrigerator until ready to serve.

6. **Dark Chocolate-Dipped Strawberries:**

   - Ingredients: Fresh strawberries, dark chocolate chips or chopped dark chocolate, coconut oil (optional), chopped nuts or shredded coconut (optional).
   - Instructions:
     1. Wash and dry the strawberries thoroughly, leaving the stems intact.
     2. In a microwave-safe bowl, melt the dark chocolate chips (or chopped dark chocolate) in 30-second intervals, stirring in between, until smooth. If desired, stir in a teaspoon of coconut oil to thin the chocolate.
     3. Dip each strawberry into the melted chocolate, coating

about two-thirds of the
berry.
4. Place the dipped
strawberries on a
parchment-lined baking
sheet.
5. Optional: Sprinkle chopped
nuts or shredded coconut on
top of the chocolate before
it sets.
6. Allow the chocolate to set at
room temperature or place
the baking sheet in the
refrigerator for quicker
setting.
7. Serve as a delightful and
indulgent treat.

CONCLUSION

As we wrap up our time together, I just want to say thank you for letting me be a part of your cooking journey. It's been great sharing these recipes with you. I hope they've brought some joy to your kitchen and maybe even inspired you to try some new things.

Cooking isn't just about food – it's about making memories and sharing moments with the people you love. I hope these recipes have helped create some special moments for you and your loved ones.

So, as you enjoy these dishes, remember the simple pleasure of good food and good company. And hey, if you ever need more recipes or cooking tips, you know where to find me! Check my Author central

Thanks again for hanging out with me in the kitchen. Take care, and happy cooking!